THE HYPNOSIS HANDBOOK

SECOND EDITION 2014

ABOUT THE AUTHOR

Dr Mark Baker is a neuroscientist and hypnotherapist specializing in, Relationship and Couple Counselling through Hypnosis and Hypnotherapy, Hypnosis and Hypnotherapy in Corporate Development and Team Building and managing the problems of Ultra High Net- Worth Individuals.

He has over 25 years of professional experience and has studied and worked at Oxford University and carried out advanced psychological research at Cambridge University in the UK.

He has published many peer-reviewed papers and presented at conferences internationally.

CONTENTS

1. INTRODUCTION TO HYPNOSIS.

I'm often asked whether there is a good book on hypnosis and while the obvious answer is "why yes, there are thousands . . .", I always pause for thought, because there are none that tell you about hypnosis in the way that I'd really like you about it.

There are technical tomes. There are volumes dripping with erudite theory. There are starry-eyed popular accounts and mystical accounts, but when it comes to simple, straightforward concise accounts for the intelligent layperson the markets seem to have a gap.

WHAT IS HYPNOSIS?

Origins: The word "hypnosis" (Greek: ὕπνωσις) comes from the Greek word hypnos, "sleep", and the suffix -osis, or from hypnoō, "(I) put to sleep" (stem of aorist hypnōs-) and the suffix -is.

Simply put, hypnosis is a mental skill in which the subject learns to control their own mental processes. They effectively learn to turn on and off parts of their own mind under the control of other parts. This might be reducing fear, they might be eliminating the negative emotions associated with certain memories, or they might be anything else that goes on in a human beings mind. More positively it might be increasing creativity, stimulating the flow of ideas or boosting happiness. This is best done under the guidance of a hypnotist or hypnotherapist. The hypnotist guides the subject into the appropriate mental state and may, in the case of great practitioners, trains them to control their own mental processes.

Once trained, many subjects can then apply these skills to themselves. By doing this they can gain extraordinary control over their own minds.

It turns out that not all hypnotists are aware of exactly what they are doing (although all have their own theories, perhaps as many as there are hypnotists) and a large proportion follow formulae passed on from books or teachers without ever being able to articulate what they are doing exactly or why. This can be a problem if they are trying to pass on the skills.

A common or garden uses of hypnosis are to allow the subject to change habits (like smoking of phobias), accommodate to mental traumas (in therapy) or – when combined with stagecraft – to provide fascinating entertainment, but this is only a tiny part of what can be achieved using hypnosis. Until you've actually experienced it, it seems like an implausible, somewhat superstitious craft. When you have experienced a hypnotic 'trance' under a good hypnotist then you begin to see that it can open up a whole new set of tools to work on your own inner processes.

This book then aims to gives you a simple, practical, common sense approach to understanding hypnosis and to being able to apply it.

2. HOW DOES HYPNOSIS WORK?

Hypnosis is usually induced by a procedure known as a hypnotic induction involving a series of preliminary instructions and suggestions

Typically the hypnotist follows a simple process of guidance giving the subject a series of instructions that the subject follows. This is called an hypnotic induction. Typically these involve getting the subject into a highly relaxed state, physically and mentally. The subject is then given instructions telling them how to clear their mind. Only the subject can do this for themselves and all hypnosis depends on the skill and participation of the subject. Once they have cleared their mind of extraneous thoughts using specific methods that the hypnotist guides them through they are able to focus their attention exclusively on the mental states that they will address with the hypnotist. A good hypnotist monitors the subject's state constantly and gives appropriate instructions to retain that focus. It is an essential part of the process that the subject follows without criticism or judgment during the process simply experiencing what happens.

James Braid, the hard-nosed, cynical Victorian Scot who set out to debunk the whole nonsense and ended up by founding the modern science of hypnosis puts it thus

"the powers of the mind are so much engrossed with a single idea or train of thought, as, for the nonce, to render the individual unconscious of, or indifferently conscious to, all other ideas, impressions, or trains of thought."

So in hypnosis, the subject learns not to let go, but to focus on a single thought or idea removing all interruptions, be they external or internal.

The words "hypnosis" and "hypnotism" both derive from the term "neuro-hypnotism" (nervous sleep) coined by the Scottish surgeon James Braid in 1841.

It's often said that Braid based his practice on that developed by Franz Mesmer and his followers but actually he has set out to debunk "Mesmerism" also known as "animal magnetism"), but found that after he had stripped away the nonsense there was still a core of material that stood up to scrutiny.

Is Hypnosis relaxation?
Again the clear-headed Braid tells us that

"The hypnotic sleep, therefore, is the very antithesis or opposite mental and physical condition to that which precedes and accompanies common sleep; for the latter arises from a diffusive state of mind, or complete loss of power of fixing the attention, with suspension of voluntary power."

Although we use normally relaxation to start the process and remove extraneous inference it is by no means essential and is the tiniest part of the journey that the subject can embark on.

IS HYPNOSIS A FORM OF MIND CONTROL?

No – definitely not. No one can make you do anything under hypnosis that you don't want to do. All the hypnotist does is to guide you. Having said that you've seen people on television and stage shows being hypnotized and acting amusingly – but that reflects an inner need of the individuals selected to perform on stage or television. Nevertheless if anyone asks you to do something that you don't want to you will snap out of hypnosis very quickly!

Official bodies certainly don't see it as mind control either. The Society for Psychological Hypnosis, which is part of the American Psychological Association (APA) the leading professional body in America, published the following formal definition of Hypnosis in 2005:

> Hypnosis typically involves an introduction to the procedure during which the subject is told that suggestions for imaginative experiences will be presented. The hypnotic induction is an extended initial suggestion for using one's imagination, and may contain further elaborations of the introduction. A hypnotic procedure is used to encourage and evaluate responses to suggestions. When using hypnosis, one person (the subject) is guided by another (the hypnotist) to respond to suggestions for changes in subjective experience,

alterations in perception, sensation, emotion, thought or behavior. Persons can also learn self-hypnosis, which is the act of administering hypnotic procedures on one's own. If the subject responds to hypnotic suggestions, it is generally inferred that hypnosis has been induced. Many believe that hypnotic responses and experiences are characteristic of a hypnotic state. While some think that it is not necessary to use the word "hypnosis" as part of the hypnotic induction, others view it as essential.

WHO DOES HYPNOSIS WORK ON?

As you might, by now, be gathering, all hypnosis is self- hypnosis. It's a skill that the subject learns and applies to themselves. The skill, empathy and methods used by the hypnotist makes a substantial difference.

Typically, however, about 20% of subjects – about one in five will go into trance easily and for just about any hypnotist, while another 20% are highly resistant and find the skill impossible to master. The other 60% - the large majority of subjects find trace possible with the correct understanding of the task (essentially the material in this section of this book) and a calm, empathic hypnotist.

Theoretical scales of hypnotic susceptibility do exist and are used in research – such as the Harvard Group Scale of Hypnotic Susceptibility and the Stanford Hypnotic

Susceptibility Scales, but these tend to use a recording to try to hypnotize the subject to remove the human factor – but in the process removing the skill and empathy from the equation.

WHAT DOES HYPNOSIS FEEL LIKE?

A person under hypnosis could be thought of as experiencing heightened focus and concentration on a specific thought or memory, while blocking out sources of distraction.

Hypnosis is a state of focused attention so it resembles other similar states that we are familiar with. When we drive across town we don't remember every gear change or every move of the steering wheel – our attention is refocused – ideally on the road and it's that which we remember – not the small actions that got us there. Likewise we regularly create vivid mental imagery in our heads when we read or hear a story without remembering the layout of the text or what is happening away from the book. These experiences are analogous to hypnosis. So typically what a subject feels is a relaxing calm and the subject is conscious throughout hearing and remembering everything. The idea of a trance that is sleep-like and amnesic is outside the usual experience. However subjects typically report a dive or swaying feeling as they change "state" and imagery and visualizations can be intense and realistic once the subject has practiced with a really good hypnotist.

The brilliant and much admired, Nobel Laureate physicist Richard Feynman, gave an excellent explanation. After describing his thoughts as he complied with a suggestion to leave his seat and walk around the auditorium, Feynman said:

"I kept asking myself why am I doing this? I knew that I didn't have to do it but somehow I just felt like doing it. I suppose that's what hypnosis is."

WHAT CAN YOU DO WITH HYPNOSIS?

Well, you can: improve social confidence; remove phobias; carry out anger management; aid weight loss; improve sports training; create altered states; fix relationships in families, couples or even companies. The more you understand about hypnosis the more you'll see that that is actually just the beginning.

If you consider that everything that you see and know about in the universe is perceived inside your head - everything you know and understand -and how you view and feel about any and all of that can be changed if you want to using hypnosis – then you can begin to understand how powerful a tool this is.

IS HYPNOSIS LIKE MEDITATION?

There is a long history of similar techniques being used for thousands of years – for example in the Patañjali, the Yoga Sutras (c. 250 B.C., § 1.34-38) we are told

> "Mental equanimity may be attained by regulating the exhalation and restraint of the breath. Or the wayward mind may be pacified by focusing attention upon a single object. [...] Alternatively, one can meditate by focusing attention upon the experience of dreaming, or the state of dreamless sleep [yoga nidra]".

However it is my experience that even highly experiences meditators with twenty years or more of experience are astonished by how effective hypnosis is in achieving a deep state and guiding the mind to new thoughts and experiences. In this sense hypnosis with a guide who really understand what they are doing (rather than a specialist who has simply learned the technology of say stopping smoking or weight loss) is an immensely effective form of guided meditation. If through mediation you are a cork bobbing in the sea, then through guided mediation and through hypnosis you are on a voyage on a great square- sailed ship across the oceans with the winds billowing in your sails and the only limits are those you choose to impose upon yourself.

3. GETTING STARTED WITH HYPNOSIS.

A common misconception is that hypnosis is a form of unconsciousness resembling sleep. In reality hypnotic subjects are fully awake and are focusing attention, with a corresponding decrease in their peripheral awareness.

Subjects also show an increased response to suggestions.

In the first ever book on the subject, "Neurypnology" published in 1843, James Braid described "hypnotism" as a state of physical relaxation accompanied and induced by mental concentration ("abstraction")

TRYING OUT YOUR FIRST HYPNOTIC INDUCTION

Unless you want to be an advanced stage hypnotist (and often even then) the Elman Induction is the only method of inducing hypnosis that you'll ever need – in much the same way that if you have a good car you'll find that generally you won't need a hovercraft or an airship or even roller-skates to get to work each day.

The Elman induction can be tried out in a few minutes. It can be learned well in a few days. Yet it is probably the most powerful way of inducing hypnosis known. It is good enough for dentists to use it to extract teeth without any other anaesthetic. It is used by midwives to use it for natural childbirth without anaesthetic. It's even been used by surgeons for procedures as invasive as heart surgery with anaesthetic.

The only reason why advanced stage hypnotists might want to try something else once they master the Elman is for the purposes of stagecraft and to give a show which is less familiar to the audience.

In the version that I use I've used my personal experience of over twenty years of advanced psychology and neuroscience and forty years of quantitative research knowledge from the publications since Elman as well as personal experience from hypnotizing hundreds of clients to further refine the excellent technique to make it easier, more foolproof and more effective. It's the difference between using a 1961 Porsche 911 and this year's top of the range model – the latter building on the success of the former and so strangely similar superficially, both superb but the newest benefiting from half a century of experience:

more refined, easier to use and ultimately faster.

So actually this is Dr Baker's version of the Elman induction. This is how it goes. You can just read it to your subject, but there are notes further on that tell you how to quickly become a real hypnotist using this script. Start from a gentle version of your own voice and slowly move to how you would talk to a sleeping child who you felt affectionate and protective about.

Do you want to be hypnotized?

Yes

Do you want to be hypnotized by me?

OK

Good.

Now for hypnosis to work we have to agree to work together.

Now your task is to follow what I say, to suspend judgment until we finish and to get into and enjoy the experience.

My task is to guide you through, take it seriously, be responsible and work my hardest to make this work. Is this all fine for you?

Yes

Just begin by making yourself comfortable. Rest your feet flat on the floor and rest your hands on your thighs.

All throughout this process if any thoughts come into your head imagine putting them in bubbles then pop the bubbles of thoughts.

If silly thoughts come into your head that's fine - put them in bubbles and pop them too - let the fun out.

And if you hear any sounds or distractions along the way just think of them as part of the experience and let them take you deeper.

Now drop your head forward slightly and roll your eyes up and back as though you were looking toward a point in your forehead.

That's a bit of a strain but keep it up. Now, inhale deeply, filling your lungs all the way up as you continue to look up and back. Pause for a few seconds. Now keep looking up and allow your eyelids to grow heavy and close down... as you exhale slowly and patiently. Good, now send a huge wave of relaxation from the top of your head down to the tip of your toes. Let all of your muscles turn loose, and limp and wonderfully relaxed... just like a rag doll. Remember, if any thoughts come into your head imagine putting them in bubbles then pop the bubbles of thoughts.

Now, rest your awareness on those eyelids once again. Even though the eyelids are closed down comfortably already, imagine they are closing down all over again, even more heavy and tired and lazy than before. Now relax those eyelids right down to the point where it feels as if they just don't work anymore. When you know you've done that, make a test and find you've succeeded and they feel as if they're sealing shut. Push harder against that relaxation and find the harder you try to make the effort the more lazy and tired and relaxed those eyelids are becoming right now. Now stop trying,

Now Dr Baker says that this is just the first step and that this is one of the most astonishing amazing things you'll ever experience

It will change your life to be immensely better and put you more in control if you let it

Just feel that happiness now and let it set in by feeling thankful about this technique [wait 20 seconds]

And as you feel that happiness again be excited to learn more. Just ask me more when you emerge [wait 10 seconds]

And as you feel that happiness again be excited to tell more friends – they are going to love it and be so pleased [wait 10 seconds]

And as you feel that happiness again be excited to try again and to plan more of this type of hypnosis into your life now. [wait 10 seconds]

In a moment I'm going to count from 1 to 5. As I count from 1 to 5 it's going to give you all the time you need to come all the way back out of trance. But as you come back out of trance [subject name], you're going to lock in these lessons and learnings. You're going to be having a wonderful time, looking forward to all the sessions we're going to have together.

If the session seems to be going well and you are both enjoying it continue otherwise simply count the subject out.

And wondering, curious, just what Dr Baker's methods can teach you this time to make your life better forever. And I want you to be totally free in your responses to me [subject name]. Because you're the one, you're the one it's all about. You're the one who gets all the benefit, and you're the one that I'm counting on, to give me as clean and pure and powerful response as you possibly can. I want you to do your best to totally open up and simply listen, accept, obey, and feel happiness, and trust that I'll lead you into a wonderful place. Because two, my suggestions and commands go in so deep they become your permanent and natural way of thinking. All my commands are murmuring away inside now helping to watch over you, protect you, and guide you, and show you the way. You love hearing my voice inside.

That's right, it makes you feel happiness in your mind and happiness in your body. And three, we're going to be exploring just how addictive happiness can be for you, so all throughout our sessions, and all through the time we spend together, you're going to feel pure, addictive happiness. That's right, binding us closer and closer together. And your eager desire to obey and be pleasing grows stronger as four, take a deep deep breath. Feel the energy returning, flowing cleanly all throughout mind and body. Feel yourself relaxed, in perfect harmony, mind, body and spirit, all attuned, that's right, you feel like you had a great, great experience, and when you open your eyes, only when I count five you'll open your eyes and return all the way back to the room.

You'll remember everything perfectly, only happy memories, realize you just had a fantastic [first] session, preparing you to work together with me over the next couple of days to explore all the ways that you can get closer, feel better, and allow me to... change you... into a better person.

That's right, you're really into this.

And five [snap], eyes open, wide awake. Wide awake feeling fantastic, and [subject name], how do you feel?

Basically if you go through this script you have a good chance of getting a hypnotic effect of some type. If you follow the other instructions in this book carefully then you'll almost certainly be able to deeply and effectively hypnotize almost anyone who wants to be hypnotized.

4. UNDERSTANDING WHAT IS HAPPENING IN HYPNOSIS.

STEP-BY-STEP GUIDANCE THROUGH THE BAKER-ELMAN INDUCTION

So here is a step-by-step breakdown of what is happening in my version of the Elman induction.

Every part counts and works with every other part.

There are over fifty years of refinements over the original Elman induction, all are individually tested over hundreds of subjects and the impact of my complete process is spectacularly improved even over Elman's impressive contribution[1]. For comparison, Elman's own original is in an appendix at the end of this book.

As I indicated before you can just read it to your subject, but if you are stumbling over the words due to not practicing you'll lack congruence (or harmony, or just getting their confidence). Nevertheless it is probably better to stumble than not do it at all. Whatever you do don't fall into the robotic toneless droning of some hypnotists – just be kind and gentle as you are asking your subject to trust you completely and if you break that trust at any stage they will just snap out, come around and probably never let you try again.

---

[1] As the undisputed greatest genius of the modern age Isaac Newton, said "If I have seen a little further it is by standing on the shoulders of Giants"

Do you want to be hypnotized? Do you
want to be hypnotized by me?

This is what we call the hypnotic contract and gets their spoken and definite permission. It's important both ethically and operationally to do this. Say this every time you hypnotize your subject.

Good.

Now for hypnosis to work we have to agree to work together. Now your task is to follow what I say, to suspend judgment until we finish and to get into and enjoy the experience. My task is to guide you through, take it seriously, be responsible and work my hardest to make this work. Is this all fine for you? You need to outline this clearly and get agreement in words. If the subject tries to lead or turns this into a battle of wills it will fail from the outset and you'll both be demoralized.

Just begin by making yourself
comfortable. Rest your feet flat on the
floor and rest your hands on your thighs.

You are aiming for (and needing) compliance and this is your first test. Did they do what you said or was there some excuse? Just explain that is the way (unless there is some real reason why they can't do this). Go back to discussing the contract if they don't follow

All throughout this process if any thoughts come into your head imagine putting them in bubbles then pop the bubbles of thoughts. If silly thoughts come into your head that's fine - put them in bubbles and pop them too - let the fun out. And if you hear any sounds or distractions along the way just think of them as part of the experience and let them take you deeper.

These are two valuable master techniques used to obtain an effective hypnotic trance. Make sure that you always do them and feel free to repeat either if it seems necessary.

Now drop your head forward slightly and roll your eyes up and back as though you were looking toward a point in your forehead. That's a bit of a strain but keep it up. Now, inhale deeply, filling your lungs all the way up as you continue to look up and back. Pause for a few seconds. Now keep looking up and allow your eyelids to grow heavy and close down... as you exhale slowly and patiently.

This is one of the oldest and most powerful methods in modern hypnosis. The change from the enforced strain (which also clears the subjects mind) to relaxation creates the first step into hypnosis. With a difficult subject (but one who will follow you) you can extend that eye-strain period out to as long as a minute or more to make then really clear their minds.

Good, now send a huge wave of relaxation from the top of your head down to the tip of your toes. Let all of your muscles turn loose, and limp and wonderfully relaxed... just like a rag doll.

Feel free to describe that relaxation spreading through their bodies (eyes, temples, forehead, mouth, tongue, neck shoulders etc). Make the voice caressing.

Be slow and gentle. Be certain not to do anything that might spoil the relaxation.

Remember, if any thoughts come into your head imagine putting them in bubbles then pop the bubbles of thoughts.

Just keep using this any time the subject seems to be starting to think of something else. This is where empathy comes in!

Now, rest your awareness on those eyelids once again. Even though the eyelids are closed down comfortably already, imagine they are closing down all over again, even more heavy and tired and lazy than before. Now relax those eyelids right down to the point where it feels as if they just don't work anymore. When you know you've done that, make a test and find you've succeeded and they feel as if they're sealing shut. Push harder against that relaxation and find the harder you try to make the effort the more lazy and tired and relaxed those eyelids are becoming right now. Now stop trying, send a wave of relaxation right down into that part of you that was trying to make the effort. You're eyelids aren't really sealed shut, it just feels as if they are. That's a good sign, you're relaxing very deeply.

This is the eyelid catalepsy test and is an excellent test of relaxation, susceptibility and willingness to co-operate with the hypnosis process. You should only to tell them to test the eyes only when you know that they have relaxed them sufficiently to not open them. You can add in a line telling them that if they can't open their eyes "that proves that they are following well". Some hypnotists get people who say, "well do you want me to open my eyes?". In that case explain to them that when the eyes get so relaxed, they get to a stage where they can't open. Their aim, then, is to can relax their eyes to that point they will NOT open.

Now, I'm going to help you to relax even more deeply, and this is how I'm going to do it. In a moment I'll count 1, 2, 3, when I reach the number three you can open your eyes for a second before I gesture and say the word "sleep." When I say the word "sleep", just allow your eyelids to close down and find you're going back, even deeper into hypnosis than before. Beginning now, 1, 2, 3... opening those eyelids, ready now, "sleep", relaxing much deeper than before, two times deeper... Good... Once again, 1, 2, 3, opening those eyelids, ready now, "sleep", relaxing much deeper than before, two times deeper... Good... One more time now, 1, 2, 3, opening those eyelids, ready now, "sleep", relaxing much deeper than before, two times deeper again... Good.

In hypnosis, this is a method of induction (Vogt's fractionation method) where the subject is partially relaxed then roused and asked to recount the sensations experienced. Then the hypnosis/relaxation continues again, often with the therapist 'feeding back' the recounted experience and leading the patient still deeper. The patient is then roused again and his experiences sought, before the hypnosis resumes once again. The process continues until a deep trance state is obtained.

This is a variation. Fractionation is based on the principle that when you take a person in and out of trance, they tend to go more deeply into trance when you take them back in. Thus when you have them open their eyes, you are breaking their state.

When you have them open their eyes, put your hand in front of their eye-lids so they don't see the lights/distractions around them ... lift your hand up a little bit for the open motion, and then guide their eyes down with the closed motion. You can use this method any time during the induction or hypnosis if you think the subject is not in a deep enough trance[2].

I'm now going to lift your hand and drop it and if you've followed orders up to this point that hand will be just as limp as a dishrag and will just plop into your lap... No, let me lift it -don't you lift it- let it be heavy - that's good- but let's open and close the eyes again and double that relaxation and send it right down to your toes. Let that hand be as heavy as lead...

[2] Of course this can't be done in larger groups

You'll feel it when you've got the real relaxation... Now you've got it. You could feel that, couldn't you?

"Yes"

This is a motor catalepsy test. You can repeat this test at random points during the hypnosis if you want to deepen the relaxation, because it is an already accepted mechanism that if you lift and drop their hand, they'll go deeper. You have to make sure that they have completely relaxed their hand and arm. You may find that it sometimes helps to give a little bit of touch around the shoulder joint because it implies that the hand is disconnected.

Now you're relaxing the body very deeply, and as you relax the body you're relaxing the mind. Now, I'm going to help you to relax the mind even more deeply and this is how I'm going to do it. In a moment I want you to begin counting down backwards from 100, counting out loud, and repeating the words "deeper and deeper" after each number. Each time you say the words "deeper and deeper", you're doubling the relaxation of your mind, especially the counting part of your mind. By the time you've counted just a few of those numbers, to 95 or even 96, you'll find you've succeeded in relaxing your mind so deeply that you just can't be bothered even trying to locate those numbers, they've vanished completely, forgotten from your mind. Start counting now, losing the numbers to relaxation as you count, beginning now...

Intersperse suggestions of deepening such as "twice as deep into hypnosis" and "that's good" until subject stops counting.

That's it. Good. Now relax even more deeply, and as you do so make an effort and try to locate those forgotten numbers and find that you've succeeded, they've faded completely from the mind. Haven't they? Make sure that you get them to say the words "deeper and deeper" in between the numbers.

For clients who might take a longer time to get the effect, this will speed up the process because they are saying "deeper relaxed" out of their own mouth."

Make sure they understand that they will count out loud, slowly, and backwards. This is very important when doing your Elman Induction. If you are in a crowded place, somewhere where they may not want to be overheard or hypnotizing a group tell the subject to mouth the number quietly.

When you tell them that by the time they reach "96 or even 97? you are telling them that the numbers will be gone quickly, and you are testing for somnambulism. If you say a lower number even though it seems like you are making it more likely that they'll get the effect, in fact they will simply take longer and the convincer aspect of it won't be there as much.

If they continue to count, you can intersperse the numbers with suggestions like: "Just make them gone now .. I can't do it for you .. If you want it, it will happen instantly" ... If they still continue to not forget the numbers (that is fail at the test) then transition to something else, as if they've done perfectly. Some people will take longer than others though. At the end, say

"All gone?" or "Are they gone?"

... Don't say "Can you see the numbers?" because that is a direct suggestion for them to see the numbers

Now I want you to fade out the parts of your mind that did the fading out. Just tune them out completely.

Now image that you open your eyes and in front of you, you see a door. You step forward and open the door and outside you see clouds. You step through and unfurl your wings and you are an Eagle soaring high above the clouds. You feel the cold wing on your wings, see the distant horizon sharply, you turn and spiral down and down becoming more and more detached from the mundane world and deeper and deeper into hypnosis . . .

repeat suggestions of "turning" and getting deeper between ten and sixty seconds . . .

This is my special hypnotic deepener. Clients report it as being much more powerful than traditional deepeners and it opens up a number of intriguing opportunities as you grow more advanced.

As you touch the ground and land you hear my voice say "sleep now" and I hypnotize you you are in a world of happiness.

You hear me ask you to think of one of the great happy feelings of your life, something you experience or would like to experience in your ideal life.

Image the feeling, smell the smells, hear the sounds, feel the touch, see the colors and shapes.

Make it real. [wait]

Can you feel that now? [wait again]

Just let it build up and let the feeling flow around your body like blood from the top of your body down to your toes. Just raise a hand when you can't feel it get any stronger.

This is the start of my unique method for creating positive resources. It's based on a method developed over 20 years ago by a senior US military hypnotist for managing combat trauma, but I've extended it and added carefully selected research-proven methods, so that anyone can use it to improve subjects overall happiness, confidence and ability to cope.

[after hand raise]

Now we are going to use the next part of Dr Baker's special technique to enhance hypnotic learning.

Imagine there is a dial inside you like a volume control or a cooker temperature dial. We both reach inside you now and turn up the dial. As we turn it your happiness gets more intense. Let's try it. Can you feel that . . .? Can you turn it up more? . . [wait] more? . . . [wait] that's great.

Over hundreds of subjects one thing that I've learned is that it is important to distinguish these techniques, my techniques, from generic hypnosis. Firstly it imparts a special focus both for the subject and the hypnotist which greatly improves outcome. But also secondarily it remove the phenomenon which is so common where subjects go away impressed and astonished and keen to learn more – and then pick up a random book on hypnosis or go to a regular therapist and after much striving, time and expense go away disheartened and demoralized , despondent that they could never reproduce the first rush that they got from my methods and techniques.

So all this is part of Dr Baker's special technique and what I want you to do now is every time you hear me say the word happiness you feel just this way.

This is setting the trigger that allows the subject to feel happiness. Use it frequently (two or three times a day), but always appropriately after hypnosis. If you overuse it or use it inappropriately then you will basically break the training as well as losing your credibility with your subject.

Now Dr Baker says that this is just the first step and that this is one of the most

astonishing, amazing things you'll ever
experience

Tell them this conversationally. They need to know that this is not all there is to it. At this particular stage they can now also reasonably believe that it is "one of the most astonishing, amazing things you'll ever experience". If you haven't experienced this yourself then you'll need to get someone to hypnotize you using my methods so that you know that it's actually true.

After the first time successfully hypnotizing your subject suggest a little game at this stage called the "tell me" game. In this they repeat the lines below back to you acting out as though they said them themselves and they are already true. This seems sort of cheesy but it's like acting and really adds to the fun that everyone gets from this.

It will change your life to be immensely
better and put you more in control if you
let it

"This will change my life to be
immensely better and put me more in
control if I let it"

44

Just feel that happiness now and let it set in by feeling thankful about this technique [wait 20 seconds]

"I feel happiness now. I feel thankful about this technique"

And as you feel that happiness again be excited to learn more. Just ask me more when you emerge [wait 10 seconds]

"I'll ask you more about this technique when I emerge"

And as you feel that happiness again be excited to tell more friends – they are going to love it and be so pleased [wait 10 seconds]

"I'm excited and going get all my friends to try this out – they are going to love it and be so pleased"

And as you feel that happiness again be excited to try again and to plan more of

this type of hypnosis into your life now.
[wait 10 seconds]

> "I'm excited and happy and going to try
> again and to plan more of this type of
> hypnosis into my life now"

In a moment I'm going to count from 1 to
5. As I count from 1 to 5 it's going to give
you all the time you need to come all the
way back out of trance. But as you come
back out of trance [subject name], you're
going to lock in these lessons and
learnings. You're going to be having a
wonderful time, looking forward to all the
sessions we're going to have together.

Probably best to stop at this stage for the first
session. If the subject seems to be really into
their hypnosis you can try this longer wind
down.

[If the session seems to be going well and you
are both enjoying it continue otherwise simply
count the subject out]

And wondering, curious, just what Dr Baker's methods can teach you this time to make your life better forever. And I want you to be totally free in your responses to me [subject name]. Because you're the one, you're the one it's all about. You're the one who gets all the benefit, and you're the one that I'm counting on, to give me as clean and pure and powerful response as you possibly can. I want you to do your best to totally open up and simply listen, accept, obey, and feel happiness, and trust that I'll lead you into a wonderful place. Because two, my suggestions and commands go in so deep they become your permanent and natural way of thinking. All my commands are murmuring away inside now helping to watch over you, protect you, and guide you, and show you the way. You love hearing my voice inside. That's right, it makes you feel happiness in your mind and happiness in your body. And three, we're going to be exploring just how addictive happiness can be for you, so all throughout our sessions, and all through the time we spend together, you're going to feel pure, addictive happiness. That's right, binding us closer and closer together. And your eager desire to obey and be pleasing grows stronger as four, take a deep deep breath. Feel the energy returning, flowing cleanly all throughout mind and body. Feel yourself relaxed, in perfect harmony, mind, body and spirit, all attuned, that's right, you feel like you had a great, great experience, and when you open your eyes, only when I count five you'll open your eyes and return all the way back to the room. You'll remember everything perfectly, only happy memories, realize you just had a fantastic [first] session, preparing you to work together with me over the next couple of days to explore all the ways that you can get closer, feel better, and allow me to... change you... into a better person. That's right, you're

> really into this. And five [snap], eyes
> open, wide awake. Wide awake feeling
> fantastic, and [subject name], how do you
> feel?

It's best to do this a few times (about six is supposed to be most effective) on each person you try it on. You can easily have a situation where it doesn't seem to be effective the first time, but after the second or third – wham – they get the point, you get the knack and it all comes together. For extra effectiveness after the first time you can get them to tell numbers 14 to 19 back to you aloud – this really speeds up the process and gets great results. In any case the effect fades in hours to a couple of days after the first time you hypnotize them but if you do it again within that time it lasts longer and longer and is stronger and stronger. If you follow these instructions carefully you'll almost certainly be able to deeply and effectively hypnotize almost anyone who wants to be hypnotized.

IMPROVING YOUR SKILLS AS A HYPNOTIST

Well there is no point in messing around - this is an amazing skill to have – actually life changing – but it really becomes tremendously rewarding when you do it properly. There are a few things that can take you from being a dabbler who says "I read a book about it once, I think it worked but I can't quite remember" to this being a key life skill like reading, driving or swimming where you've always got something to fall back on if you or a friend feels stressed or depressed and you've always got something that makes you the most fascinating person in the room at parties or with new friends. Read and do what's in this chapter and you'll be the latter instead of the former.

TALKING THE TALK

The simplest thing to do is to practice the Elman script by reading it aloud before you read it to someone as part of a hypnosis. Even better I suggest you do is to read it to your Smartphone and record yourself reading it. Don't forget to speak gently as if to a child who is not well. You don't even need to listen to yourself after – but do it as if it's for real – with feeling and expression. If you can do this half a dozen times you'll be astonished how much better you'll get and how professional people will think you sound. Really!

EDUCATING YOUR SUBJECTS

Educated subjects are much, much, much more receptive and improve your success rate from 20% (one in five) to 80% (four in five). This one is a no brainer. It's simple. Just suggest that they read this book. This isn't a cheap marketing ploy – short of working with a first rate hypnotist for half a day the best way of getting your subject to improve their hypnotic skills that I know of is to read this book. That's why I wrote it.

WALKING THE WALK

Well not literally! However, the next level beyond being really practiced, the thing that allows you to do this in a pub, a party or if a friend is feeling low, and to do it well, without looking like an amateur, is to memorize my version of the Elman Induction. This is easier than it sounds if you use this old memory system. What you need to do is take your Baker-Elman Script on a familiar journey with you. Maybe to work or to the local shops. At each step of the journey read part of the script and imagine a comic, over-exaggerated version of that step associated with that place. So you are sitting comfortably with bubbles popping around your head on your from doorstep. Then you are walking down your street (see the picture of walking down the street with your eyes rolled right back holding your breath). Image this (or better do this) a few times, saying the right part of the script at the right times and you'll find it easy to remember. This works really well if you try it and is a fun and painless way to remember. Now you are going to actually look like a cool hypnotist and you can use the method at a party, on a date, on the bus (or your Learjet) or when conversation gets dull.

GOING LIVE

You'll find that your hypnotic skills really take off after you've tried this a bit on real people in the real world. Don't be shy - I suggest that you try this out on about six different friends, colleagues or acquaintances. Try it a few times on each one. If you are social then you could be trying this almost every day for a month and finding it more fun and more interesting. It's actually a good ice breaker and way of meeting new people "I was reading this really interesting book about psychology the other day". A few subjects are going to be less helpful than others – try it on easy, friendly amenable ones first. After about half a dozen people you'll be astonished how good you are going to be at this and how impressed people will be.

But don't let any of this stop you

But don't let any of this stop you – it's better to just try it out than to be put off by the need to get it all right! Just do it!

5. SELF HYPNOSIS

So the obvious question is – can I use hypnosis to improve my life? Well, the answer is, yes, profoundly!

Here is what to do. You'll see as you read later that Home Study Self-Hypnosis has approximately a 2 – 5% success rate – compared with 85 – 90% success rate for five or more individual sessions with an expert hypnotist. This really explains why everyone doesn't use hypnosis themselves to improve their lives. On the other hand lots of highly successful people attribute success to hypnosis. So what is the reason for this apparent contradiction? It's simple really. It's a question of how you were trained and how closely the hypnotic materials that you used matched your own particular needs.

So it falls into two parts

To be effective in self hypnosis you need to really be trained to be hypnotized and learn all the hypnotic skills. Ideally you learn from an expert – it typically takes about half a dozen sessions to get really good. Failing that either way you must start with general hypnotic training rather than just using a recording labelled "the Perfect Hypnosis Download" or

"Gain Confidence". But here is the good news. All you really need to do is make yourself a recording of the Elman induction in this book exactly as it is and play it back to yourself every day for a couple of weeks, being the subject yourself. Don't forget to do the "tell me" too, even if you just mouth the words. Then you can move on to add suggestions to the later part of the process and make a new recording. Of course this can never be as effective as hypnosis under a master hypnotist – but it's going to be tremendously more effective than any generic bought-in hypnosis recording and you are going to end up with the best self-hypnosis recording for yourself.

Dr Baker's Tricks of the Trade

Dr Baker's useful phases that can be added in anytime anywhere.

If you need to get the subject out of trance fast(emergency only)

"When I clap my hands you come back full alert - ten times more alert and awake than ever before."

If things don't seem to be going well (normally don't give up – but this is your exit if you have to)

"That's fine - now on the count of three I'm going to let you come back - three, two, one, open your eyes . . ."

If the subject looks confused (you can tell them this before as well)

"If you are confused or don't hear don't worry just go along and fill it in for yourself."

If the subject looks as though they might be thinking of something else

"If any thoughts come into your head imagine putting them in bubbles then pop the bubbles of thoughts. "

If the subject looks as though they might be thinking of something else amusing

If silly thoughts come into your head that's fine - put them in bubbles and pop them too - let the fun out.

Also

Each smile [giggle] sends you deeper into hypnosis.

If something is happening that might distract the subject (e.g. a siren or voices)

And if you hear any sounds or distractions along the way just think of them as part of the experience and let them take you deeper.

WHAT IF MY SUBJECT IS TOO STRESSED TO HYPNOTIZE?

Sometimes subjects claim to be too stressed to be hypnotized or just seem too agitated to do anything useful. If they are this is a simple but powerful exercise based on the Buddhist disciple of mindfulness of thoughts. Mindfulness might simply be described as choosing and learning to control our focus of attention. Mindfulness does not conflict with any beliefs or tradition, religious, cultural or scientific. It is simply a practical way to notice thoughts, physical sensations, sights, sounds, smells - anything we might not normally notice. The actual skills are very simple. Just lead your subject through the exercise reading the word below you start any hypnosis.

"LEAVES ON A STREAM" EXERCISE

Sit in a comfortable position and either close your eyes or rest them gently on a fixed spot in the room.

Visualize yourself sitting beside a gently flowing stream with leaves floating along the surface of the water. Pause 10 seconds.

58

For the next few minutes, take each thought that enters your mind and place it on a leaf... let it float by. Do this with each thought – pleasurable, painful, or neutral. Even if you have joyous or enthusiastic thoughts, place them on a leaf and let them float by.

If your thoughts momentarily stop, continue to watch the stream. Sooner or later, your thoughts will start up again. Pause 20 seconds.

Allow the stream to flow at its own pace. Don't try to speed it up and rush your thoughts along. You're not trying to rush the leaves along or "get rid" of your thoughts. You are allowing them to come and go at their own pace.

 If your mind says "This is dumb," "I'm bored," or "I'm not doing this right" place those thoughts on leaves, too, and let them pass. Pause 20 seconds.

If a leaf gets stuck, allow it to hang around until it's ready to float by. If the thought comes up again, watch it float by another time. Pause 20 seconds.

If a difficult or painful feeling arises, simply acknowledge it. Say to yourself, "I notice myself having a feeling of boredom/impatience/frustration." Place those thoughts on leaves and allow them float along.

From time to time, your thoughts may hook you and distract you from being fully present in this exercise. This is normal. As soon as you realize that you have become sidetracked, gently bring your attention back to the visualization exercise.

For any excessively stressed subject do this first before attempting hypnosis using the Elman induction.

THREE THINGS YOU SHOULD NEVER DO.

Hypnosis is a tremendously powerful method and the techniques that you already know from using this book give you tremendous powers and responsibility once you master them. So there are a few things that you need to know.

Don't tamper with memories unless you are highly trained and skilled except to remove recent minor issues that you subject agrees to let you work on. The tools and approach that you have here are already far more powerful than those used by many therapists and it is best to use them to educate your friends and acquaintances about what can be done before referring them to an expert using these particular techniques. You CAN change and remove memories using these techniques – but you are not a therapist at this stage. Many therapists will give a 10% referral fee so don't worry about losing out financially, but really a good therapist is not motivated by money – but by definition a professional does need it to make a living.

Don't regress to earlier parts of a person's life unless you are trained to. As well as the risk changing memories, you may unearth early traumatic incidents which you are not currently trained to handle. These can cause abreactions, a type of catharsis, which you can Google, but fall outside the scope of this book.

Don't try to control anyone against their will or make them do anything they might not want to do. This isn't Jedi mind control and unlike popular films or stage shows this is not going to work. Stage shows are using stage craft and books and films about this are simply fiction. What will actually happen is that your subject will "pop out" of hypnosis and since they are in a heightened, focused mental state they are going to be very displeased with you.

6. GETTING REAL FUN OUT OF HYPNOSIS.

WHAT TO DO NEXT?

As I say, I honestly suggest that you try this out on about six different friends as soon as you can. If you are social then you could be trying this almost every day for a month and finding it more fun and more interesting. Just do it!

Once you've done it on a few friends you can try groups of friends – the principle is the same but you can't do the catalepsy test and you have to pace your progress to the slowest member. Weed out trouble makers or people not taking it seriously and try to do them individually first of all.

When you've got this really working well you can try adding suggestions for what you want to achieve. You can, for example, make suggestion to your subject to make them thin or make them sleep better or make them Confident. In fact anything that is inside their head can be improved and made to work just as they want it to. You can certainly remove stress or negative feelings as well as any bocks that are allowing them to experience happiness or pleasure or any self imposed limits or unwanted behaviors. If, for example, your subject wants to learn to reduce fear and desperation and increase confidence and motivation to go for what they truly want in life, now you can help them!

The first thing to do before you start is to get them to agree in words that they want to do this. Get them to jot down what the goals are, how long they have affected them and how they affect their life. Check that they can commit at least six sessions of 90 minutes in the next month or so. Ideally in the next week. When they have done that get them to read this book. That is going to be important to their success and yours as it moves the odds in your favor from 20% to 80% if you do everything else that I outline. Now let's look at what you can do.

HOW TO MAKE HYPNOTIC SUGGESTIONS

For most people hypnosis, separates into two parts: "trance" which we have covered with the Elman Induction and suggestion. As we've seen "trance" comes about via the process of a hypnotic induction—essentially instructing and suggesting to the subject that they will enter a hypnotic state. Once a subject enters hypnosis, the hypnotist gives suggestions that can produce sought effects. Typically hypnotists will suggest things like the subject's arm is getting lighter and floating up in the air, or that a fly is buzzing around one's head. The "classic" response to an accepted suggestion that one's arm is beginning to float in the air is that the subject perceives the intended effect as happening involuntarily.

Contemporary hypnotism uses a variety of suggestion forms including direct verbal suggestions, "indirect" verbal suggestions such as requests or insinuations, metaphors and other rhetorical figures of speech, and non-verbal suggestion in the form of mental imagery, voice tonality, and physical manipulation.

Direct hypnotic suggestions are more likely to be phrased as questions or statements such as "You are a loving caring person who respects others. You respect for others is a reflection of the respect you show for yourself. You show respect for yourself in the way you dress, in the way you always take care to look your best, in the way you greet everyone with a warm and genuine smile....." etc. Indirect suggestions are less blunt than direct suggestions. For example to implant 'self respect' with an indirect suggestion you could say "I wonder if you are aware of just how much other people respect you?". The choice of suggestions is pretty much up to you but do read the section in this book on what not to do before trying them.

A distinction is commonly made between suggestions delivered "permissively" and those delivered in a more "authoritarian" manner. If you are trying to change behaviour or ways of acting suggestions are usually posthypnotic ones that are intended to trigger responses affecting behaviour for periods ranging from days to a lifetime in duration. These suggestions are often repeated in multiple sessions before they achieve peak effectiveness.

Remember that suggestions are more effective the more times they are repeated. The same suggestion can be restated in different words, or repeated in different sections of the session. A suggestion cannot be repeated too often. And always use positive wording. The wording must invoke an image of what the client wants, not what they don't want. Always end with outlining the goal and adding the suggestion "change all thoughts necessary to make it true for you". Always add the suggestion (ideally changing the wording) that this type of hypnosis is working for them and that they enjoy it.

HOW TO CREATE HYPNOTIC VISUALIZATIONS

A lot is said about hypnotic suggestions but perhaps even more than suggestions, hypnotic visualizations are a key tool in hypnosis. For example you can get your subject to visualize an ideal outcome such as a slimmer self or a group of colleagues praising them after a difficult presentation or good piece of work. Let the subject fill in the details rather than doing it yourself. Remember that the visualization should be as realistic as the subject can make it, but it doesn't have to be perfect. Your subject can fill in or correct details later. The way each person's mind works is in perfect sync with the way in which they visualizes. And the great thing is that under hypnosis their mind treats all their visualizations and imaginings as potentially real.

Having said that, get your subject to put feelings into visualizing. Incorporating the appropriate feeling into each visualization is critically important. For instance, if you want your subject to feel relaxed and confident in relation to a specific event where they normally might feel stressed, get them to imagine the event in their mind and practice feeling relaxed and confident. Repeat the visualization till they begin to naturally feel relaxed and confident any time you think of the event or a similar event or situation. And it's important for the subject to believe in what they are visualizing. This is important for achieving success with hypnosis. Tell the subject to make their visualizations seem as real as possible. Make them seem as if they are already happening.

How to Carry Out Hypnotic Training

And finally – and this is often not fully grasped by hypnotists who spend their time hopefully issuing orders to the "unconscious" – training under hypnosis matters. Use visualization to repeatedly train your subject. This is a more advanced skill and needs careful thought, but is a key to lasting success. So while you can let your subject imagine their great successes on the tennis court and that will help with confidence, using hypnosis to focus 100% on the serve that the tennis pro has been trying to coach them in and mentally rehearsing it tens and then hundreds of times will pay far greater dividends on the court.

Get your Subject to Act on Your Hypnotic Training.

If we're looking to change behavioral patterns after hypnosis we need to go out and seek opportunities to try out what has been practiced as quickly and frequently as is possible in the real world. Otherwise not only do the skills fade quickly if they are not set in by real action, but your mind soon learns not to take what you learn under hypnosis as real and relevant and it begins to be treated as a game or day-dream.

7. AFTERWORD

There are many other things that can be achieved that fall outside the scope of this book. They include: improving relationships – within couples, families or even companies; Improving Creativity; Channeling Stress and many, many more things as well as techniques such as time dilation, dissociation, imaginary lives, and adding Kino & Eye contact to your hypnosis skills. If you want to know more about these or to receive occasional free audio files that supplement this training just contact me on hypnosishandbook@gmail.com

8. APPENDICES

Frequently Asked Questions about Hypnosis

Q: Does Hypnosis work?

A: Success rates can be between 85% and 90%+ better than CBT or traditional techniques.

Dr Alfred A. Barrios (1970) conducted a longitudinal survey of the psychotherapeutic literature and discovered the following success rates for hypnotherapy versus therapeutic methods:

Psychoanalysis: 38% recovery after 600 sessions Behavior Therapy: 72% recovery after 22 sessions Hypnotherapy: 93% recovery after 6 sessions

American Society of Clinical Hypnosis reports the following success rates.:

Home Study Self-Hypnosis : 2 – 5% success rate Group Hypnosis Session: 2 – 5% success rate Single Individual Session: 17 – 20% success rate Three Individual Sessions: 45 – 50% success rate Five or More Individual Sessions: 85 – 90% success rate

The researchers also discovered that customizing and individualizing the sessions increased the effectiveness of the sessions dramatically.

Q: Isn't this all just quackery?

A: Typically sceptics tend to mix actual clinical hypnotherapy practice with other unrelated processes, new age myths, discredited techniques, stage shows or mesmerism and then proceed to criticize those practices as clinical hypnotherapy. This doesn't really constitute clear analytical thinking. In fact there are over 150,000 peer-reviewed scientific medical publications by doctors, psychologists and scientists supporting hypnosis. Don't just say "I saw something on the Internet that says that it's scientific". You can actually search and see for yourself the huge amount of ongoing scientific work based around the subject. The British Psychological Society say that hypnotherapy brings together a range of psychotherapeutic techniques that can assist with personal development, emotional difficulties and some health conditions. The British Medical Association specifically values and identifies hypnotherapy as the treatment of choice in many cases. Their findings have been published in the BMJ, under the title "Medical use of Hypnotism". So it's really no more quackery or humbug than any other branch of medicine.

Q: Will I be under your control?

A: Contrary to a popular misconception—that hypnosis is a form of unconsciousness resembling sleep—contemporary research suggests that hypnotic subjects are fully awake and are focusing attention, with a corresponding decrease in their peripheral awareness. In the first book on the subject, Neurypnology (1843), Braid described "hypnotism" as a state of physical relaxation accompanied and induced by mental concentration ("abstraction").!

Q: You say hypnosis can only affect my own mind. How can hypnosis affect problems which are in my every day life?

A: What you are really reacting to in "real life" is your own mental "map" of the world. The world and the people in it don't cause reactions in you ("he made me do it") - your brain creates a mental model of the world that your mind reacts to. But the map is just a map, not the territory itself. Changing how you read the mental model is key to any effective therapy and hypnotherapy gives the most powerful tool to changing not just the reactions but the map itself.

Q: Will I be made to cluck like a chicken or bark like a dog.?

A: The short answer is, only if that what you really want to do. Despite fiction and stage-shows hypnosis can only work with your mind - you are normally aware of everything that happens and can stop everything any time they want to although in therapy that would disrupt the therapeutic process.

Q: If it works, why don't hypnotists control the world?

A: Again, it's important to understand that clients need to work with the hypnotist and are normally aware of everything that happens. They can stop everything any time they want. When it comes to self-hypnosis the story is different and when you really dig deep with research it turns out that almost all self-made extremely successful and powerful people use processes similar to hypnosis to control their emotions and maximize their mental abilities.

Q: Is Hypnosis to do in some way with Reiki/Crystal

Healing/Light Healing/Mystism/Freud/Astrology?

A: No - although anyone can invent a mystical system and use hypnosis (and other elements of human psychology) to give it the appearance of inner power and insights in much the same way that anyone can make a cardboard monster and give it the appearance of life by adding motors, loud speakers and flashing lights. The more feeble minded skeptic might then conclude that motors, loud speakers and flashing lights are not real because the monster was not. This conclusion doesn't really depend on which systems you think are bogus and which are real.

Q: If it's real why don't doctors & dentists practice it as part of their normal service?

A: Many do, but hypnosis is time consuming and while most people can follow a process to get subjects into a hypnotic state with just a few weeks of practice and achieve things like pain relief, getting really first class results is complex and extensively skill based!

Q: Will I be made to re-live past lives?

A: It you like. Or you could be Frodo Baggins, Cleopatra or Neytiri or anyone else you like if you want to have a deep, rich intense imaginal experience under hypnosis (which is what really happens with past life regression).

Q: Will I be made to re-live early traumatic experiences?

A: No. That approach stems from what Sigmund Freud (1856–1939) developed as psychodynamics to describe the processes of the mind as flows of psychological energy (Libido). All modern research shows that this doesn't get to the root of the problems, but can plant damaging false memories . But see the next answer for the good news.

Q: Can hypnosis be used to change my memories?

A: It can and it's important not to make changes by accident as many early therapists did. If it is part of the treatment required it can be done, but we need to be careful to make any changes highly beneficial (Fleming et al 1992, Nelson 1992). This is slightly different from a technique called memory harvesting which is used allowing positive emotions from the past to be remembered better to be part of your current life story and be enhanced.

Q: Can you change my luck, my self image, my happiness, how I'm treated by others?

A: Yes, yes, yes and yes. The good news is that all those are due to your own mental mapping and the way you see events and react to them. The bad news is that if those were bad before then that means that they are all probably your own fault. But the good news is - you can change that now and choosing to do that will be your own doing too! (Wiseman 2003, 2004a, 2004b)

Classic Inductions: James Braid's Original Hypnotic Induction

James Braid's Original Eye-Fixation Hypnotic Induction Method

Take any bright object (e.g. a lancet case) between the thumb and fore and middle fingers of the left hand; hold it from about eight to fifteen inches from the eyes, at such position above the forehead as may be necessary to produce the greatest possible strain upon the eyes and eyelids, and enable the patient to maintain a steady fixed stare at the object.

The patient must be made to understand that he is to keep the eyes steadily fixed on the object, and the mind riveted on the idea of that one object. It will be observed, that owing to the consensual adjustment of the eyes, the pupils will be at first contracted: They will shortly begin to dilate, and, after they have done so to a considerable extent, and have assumed a wavy motion, if the fore and middle fingers of the right hand, extended and a little separated, are carried from the object toward the eyes, most probably the eyelids will close involuntarily, with a vibratory motion.

If this is not the case, or the patient allows the eyeballs to move, desire him to begin anew, giving him to understand that he is to allow the eyelids to close when the fingers are again carried towards the eyes, but that the eyeballs must be kept fixed, in the same position, and the mind riveted to the one idea of the object held above the eyes. In general, it will be found, that the eyelids close with a vibratory motion, or become spasmodically close

CLASSIC INDUCTIONS: DAVE ELMAN'S ORIGINAL INDUCTION

Full transcript from H. Larry Elman, son of Dave Elman, the "process steps" of the Elman induction are:

Catalepsy of Group of Small Muscles by Suggestion

Relaxation Suggestions

Fractionation

Catalepsy of Group of Large Muscles by Suggestion Amnesia

Further Deepener to Maintain Somnambulism

Rapid Induction

"Will you just take a good long deep breath and close your eyes. Now relax the muscles around your eyes to the point where those eye muscles won't work and when you're sure they won't work, test them and make sure they won't work... [Subject opens their eyes.] No, you're making sure they will work. Relax them to the point where they will not work and when you're sure they won't work, test them. Test them hard. Get complete relaxation in those muscles around the eyes... [Client now exhibits eyelid catalepsy.] Now let that feeling of relaxation go right down to your toes... In just a moment we're going to do this again and when we do it the second time you're going to be able to relax ten times as much as you're relaxed already.

"Now open your eyes. Close your eyes. Completely relax - let yourself be covered with a blanket of relaxation. Now the third time we do it you'll be able to double the relaxation which you have. Open your eyes -now relax. I'm now going to lift your hand and drop it and if you've followed orders up to this point that hand will be just as limp as a dishrag and will just plop into your lap... No, let me lift it -don't you lift it- let it be heavy -that's good- but let's open and close the eyes again and double that relaxation and send it right down to your toes. Let that hand be as heavy as lead... You'll feel it when you've got the real relaxation... Now you've got it. You could feel that, couldn't you? (Patient: Yes.)"

Deepening

"That's complete physical relaxation, but I want to show you how you can get mental relaxation as well as physical, so I'm going to ask you to start counting -when I tell you to- from a hundred backwards. Each time you say a number, double your relaxation, and by the time you get down to ninety-eight you'll be so relaxed there won't be any more numbers... Start with the idea of making that happen and watch it happen. Count out loud please. (Patient: One hundred.) Double your relaxation and watch the numbers start disappearing. (Ninety-nine.) Watch the numbers start disappearing. (Ninety-eight.) Now they'll be gone... Make it happen. You've got to do it, I can't do it. Make them disappear, dispel them, make them vanish. Are they all gone? [The subject says "yes" but on questioning and testing Elman finds that he is simply "too darn tired" to continue.]"

"So make those numbers completely disappear... Banish them... Are they gone? (No.) Make them disappear. I'm going to lift your hand and drop it, and when I do, the rest of those numbers will drop out. Want them to drop out and watch them go... Gone? (Yes.)" (Elman, Hypnotherapy, 1964: 60-65)

9. REFERENCES & READING

Barrios, Alfred A. "Hypnotherapy: A reappraisal." Psychotherapy: Theory, Research & Practice 7.1 (1970): 2.

Braid, James. Neurypnology; or, the rationale of nervous sleep, considered in relation with animal magnetism. 1843.

BMJ "Medical Use of Hypnotism." British medical journal 1.5033 (1957)

Coué, Émile, and Jean Thuillier. La maîtrise de soi-même par l'autosuggestion consciente. [Société lorraine de psychologie appliquée] E. Coué, 1925.

Elman, Dave. Hypnotherapy. Glendale. (1964). Elman, Dave. Hypnotherapy. Westwood Pub., (1970).

Fleming, Karen, Rebecca Heikkinen, and E. Thomas Dowd. "Cognitive therapy: The repair of memory." Journal of Cognitive Psychotherapy 6.3 (1992): 155-173.

Freud, Sigmund. "The standard edition of the complete psychological works of Sigmund Freud (Vol. 14)." London: Vintage (1915).

Garver, Richard B., G. Dwayne Fuselier, and Thomas B. Booth. "The hypnotic treatment of amnesia in an air force basic trainee." American Journal of Clinical Hypnosis 24.1 (1981): 3-6.

Harris, Russ. ACT made simple: An easy-to-read primer on acceptance and commitment therapy. New Harbinger Publications, 2009.

Nelson, Katherine. "Emergence of autobiographical memory at age 4." Human Development 35.3 (1992): 172- 177.

The Yoga-system of Patañjali: Or, The Ancient Hindu Doctrine of Concentration of Mind, Embracing the Mnemonic Rules, Called Yoga-sūtras of Patañjali and the Comment, Called Yoga-bhāshya, Attributed to Veda-Vyāsa and the Explanation, Called Tattva-vāicaradī, of Vāchaspati-Micra. Vol. 17. Motilal Banarsidass Publishe, 1914.

Tatia, Tukaram, ed. The Yoga Philosophy: Being the Text of Patanjali, with BhojaRajah's Commentary. Theosophical Society, 1882.

Weitzenhoffer, Andre M., and Ernest R. Hilgard. Stanford hypnotic susceptibility scale. Palo Alto, CA: Consulting Psychologists Press, 1962.

Wiseman, Richard. "The Luck Factor: The Four Essential Principles." New York: Miramax (2003).

Wiseman, Richard. The luck factor: The scientific study of the lucky mind. Random House, 2004.

Wiseman, Richard, and Caroline Watt. "Measuring superstitious belief: Why lucky charms matter." Personality and Individual Differences 37.8 (2004): 1533-1541.

Shor, Ronald E., and Emily Carota Orne. "Norms on the Harvard group scale of hypnotic susceptibility, form A." International Journal of Clinical and Experimental Hypnosis 11.1 (1963): 39-47.